Mediterranean Dash Diet Cookbook for Your Lunch & Dinner

Enjoy These Amazing Mediterranean Dash Diet Recipes for Daily Healthy Meals

Kathyrn Solano

Table of contents

5

BREAKFAST & LUNCH

Mediterranean Breakfast Salad

Servings: 2

Cooking Time: 10 Minutes

Ingredients:

4 eggs (optional)

10 cups arugula

1/2 seedless cucumber, chopped

1 cup cooked quinoa, cooled

1 large avocado

1 cup natural almonds, chopped

1/2 cup mixed herbs like mint and dill, chopped

2 cups halved cherry tomatoes and/or heirloom tomatoes cut into wedges

Extra virgin olive oil

1 lemon

Sea salt, to taste

Freshly ground black pepper, to taste

Directions:

Cook the eggs by soft-boiling them - Bring a pot of water to a boil, then reduce heat to a simmer. Gently lower all the eggs into water and allow them to simmer for 6 minutes. Remove the eggs from water and run cold water on top to stop the cooking, process set aside and peel when ready to use

In a large bowl, combine the arugula, tomatoes, cucumber, and quinoa

Divide the salad among 2 containers, store in the fridge for 2 days

To Serve: Garnish with the sliced avocado and halved egg, sprinkle herbs and almonds over top. Drizzle with olive oil, season with salt and pepper, toss to combine. Season with more salt and pepper to taste, a squeeze of lemon juice, and a drizzle of olive oil

Nutrition Info: Per Serving: Calories:2;Carbs: 18g;Total Fat: 16g;Protein: 10g

Breakfast Carrot Oatmeal

Servings: 2

Cooking Time: 10 Minutes

Ingredients:

1 cup steel-cut oats

1/2 cup raisins

1/2 tsp ground nutmeg

1/2 tsp ground cinnamon

2 carrots, grated

2 cups of water

2 cups unsweetened almond milk

1 tbsp honey

Directions:

Spray instant pot from inside with cooking spray.

Add all ingredients into the instant pot and stir well.

Seal pot with lid and cook on high for 10 minutes.

Once done, release pressure using quick release. Remove lid.

Stir and serve.

Nutrition Info: Calories: 3;Fat: 6.6 g; Carbohydrates: 73.8 g; Sugar: 33.7 g; Protein: 8.1 g; Cholesterol: 0 mg

Mediterranean Quinoa And Feta Egg Muffins

Servings: 12

Cooking Time: 30 Minutes

Ingredients:

8 eggs

1 cup cooked quinoa

1 cup crumbled feta cheese

1/4 tsp salt

2 cups baby spinach finely chopped

1/2 cup finely chopped onion

1 cup chopped or sliced tomatoes, cherry or grape tomatoes

1/2 cup chopped and pitted Kalamata olives

1 tbsp chopped fresh oregano

2 tsp high oleic sunflower oil plus optional extra for greasing muffin tins

Directions:

Pre-heat oven to 350 degrees F .

Prepare 1silicone muffin holders on a baking sheet, or grease a 12-cup muffin tin with oil, set aside.

In a skillet over medium heat, add the vegetable oil and onions, sauté for 2 minutes.

Add tomatoes, sauté for another minute, then add spinach and sauté until wilted, about 1 minute.

Remove from heat and stir in olives and oregano, set aside.

Place the eggs in a blender or mixing bowl and blend or mix until well combined.

Pour the eggs in to a mixing bowl (if you used a blender) then add quinoa, feta cheese, veggie mixture, and salt, and stir until well combined.

Pour mixture in to silicone cups or greased muffin tins, dividing equally, and bake for 30 minutes, or until eggs have set and muffins are a light golden brown.

Allow to cool completely.

Distribute among the containers, store in fridge for 2-3 days.

To Serve: Heat in the microwave for 30 seconds or until slightly heated through

Recipe Notes: Muffins can also be eaten cold. For the quinoa, I recommend making a large batch \'7b2 cups water per each cup of dry, rinsed quinoa\'7d and saving the extra for leftovers.

Nutrition Info: Calories:1Total Carbohydrates: 5g; Total Fat: 7g; Protein: 6g

Blueberry Greek Yogurt Pancakes

Servings: 6

Cooking Time: 15 Minutes

Ingredients:

1 1/4 cup all-purpose flour

2 tsp baking powder

1 tsp baking soda

1/4 tsp salt

1/4 cup sugar

3 eggs

3 tbsp vegan butter unsalted, melted

1/2 cup milk

1 1/2 cups Greek yogurt plain, non-fat

1/2 cup blueberries optional

Toppings:

Greek yogurt

Mixed berries – blueberries, raspberries and blackberries .

Directions:

In a large bowl, whisk together the flour, salt, baking powder and baking soda

In a separate bowl, whisk together butter, sugar, eggs, Greek yogurt, and milk until the mixture is smooth.

Then add in the Greek yogurt mixture from step to the dry mixture in step 1, mix to combine, allow the patter to sit for 20 minutes to get a smooth texture – if using blueberries fold them into the pancake batter.

Heat the pancake griddle, spray with non-stick butter spray or just brush with butter

Pour the batter, in 1/4 cupful's, onto the griddle.

Cook until the bubbles on top burst and create small holes, lift up the corners of the pancake to see if they're golden browned on the bottom.

With a wide spatula, flip the pancake and cook on the other side until lightly browned.

Distribute the pancakes in among the storage containers, store in the fridge for 3 day or in the freezer for 2 months.

To Serve: Reheat microwave for 1 minute (until 80% heated through) or on the stove top, drizzle warm syrup on top, scoop of Greek yogurt, and mixed berries (including blueberries, raspberries, blackberries) .

Nutrition Info: Calories:258;Total Carbohydrates: 33g;Total Fat: 8g;Protein: 11g

Vegetable Breakfast Bowl

Servings: 2

Cooking Time: 5 Minutes .

Ingredients:

Breakfast Bowl:

1 ½ cups cooked quinoa

1 lb asparagus[1], cut into bite-sized pieces, ends trimmed and discarded

1 tbsp avocado oil or olive oil

3 cups shredded kale leaves

1 batch lemony dressing

3 cups shredded, uncooked Brussels sprouts

1 avocado, peeled, pitted and thinly-sliced

4 eggs, cooked to your preference (optional)

Garnishes:

Toasted sesame seeds

Crushed red pepper

Sunflower seeds

Sliced almonds

Hummus

Lemon Dressing:

2 tsp Dijon mustard

1 garlic clove, minced

2 tbsp avocado oil or olive oil

2 tbsp freshly-squeezed lemon juice

Salt, to taste

Freshly-cracked black pepper, to taste

Directions:

In a large sauté pan over medium-high heat, add the oil

Once heated, add the asparagus and sauté for 4-5 minutes, stirring occasionally, until tender. Remove from heat and set side

Add the Brussels sprouts, quinoa, and cooked asparagus, and toss until combined .

Distribute among the container, store in fridge for 2-3 days.

To serve: In a large, mixing bowl combine the kale and lemony dressing. Use your fingers to massage the dressing into the kale for 2-3 minutes, or until the leaves are dark and softened, set aside. In a small mixing bowl, combine the avocado, lemon juice, dijon mustard, garlic clove, salt, and pepper. Assemble the bowls by smearing a spoonful of hummus along the side of each bowl, then portion the kale salad evenly between the four bowls. Top with the avocado slices, egg, and your desired garnishe.

Recipe Note: Feel free to sub the asparagus with your favorite vegetable(s), sautéing or roasting them until cooked.

Nutrition Info: Calories:632;Carbs: 52g;Total Fat: 39g;Protein: 24g

LUNCH AND DINNER RECIPES

Mediterranean Pasta Salad

Servings: 8
Cooking Time: 25 Minutes

Ingredients:
Salad:
8 oz pasta, I used farfalle, any smallish pasta works great!
1 cup rotisserie chicken, chopped
1/2 cup sun-dried tomatoes packed in oil, drained and coarsely chopped
1/2 cup jarred marinated artichoke hearts, drained and coarsely chopped
1/2 of 1 full English cucumber, chopped
1/3 cup kalamata olives, coarsely chopped
2 cups lightly packed fresh arugula
1/4 cup fresh flat leaf Italian parsley, coarsely chopped
1 small avocado, pit removed and coarsely chopped
1/3 cup feta cheese
Dressing:
4 tbsp red wine vinegar
1 ½ tbsp
dijon mustard, do not use regular mustard

1/2 tsp dried oregano

1 tsp dried basil

1 clove garlic, minced

1-2 tsp honey

1/2 cup olive oil

3 tbsp freshly squeezed lemon juice

Fine sea salt, to taste

Freshly cracked pepper, to taste

Directions:

Prepare the pasta according to package directions until al dente, drain the pasta and allow it to completely cool to room temperature, then add it to a large bowl

Add in the chopped rotisserie chicken, chopped cucumber, coarsely chopped kalamata olives, coarsely chopped sun-dried tomatoes, coarsely chopped artichoke hearts, arugula, and parsley, toss

Distribute the salad among the containers, store for 2-days

Prepare the dressing - In a mason jar with a lid, combine the red wine vinegar, Dijon mustard, garlic, 1/2 teaspoon salt (or to taste), dried oregano, dried basil and 1/teaspoon pepper (or to taste, honey (add to sweetness preference), olive oil, and freshly squeezed lemon juice, place the lid on the mason jar and shake to combine, store in fridge

To Serve: Add in the avocado and feta cheese to the salad, drizzle with the dressing, adjust any seasonings salt and pepper to taste, serve

Nutrition Info: Calories:32Carbs: 24g; Total Fat: 21g; Protein: 8g

Lemon Herb Avocado Chicken Salad

Servings: 4

Cooking Time: 15 Minutes

Ingredients:

Marinade/ Dressing:

2 tbsp olive oil

1/4 cup fresh lemon juice

2 tbsp water

2 tbsp fresh chopped parsley

2 tsp garlic, minced

1 tsp each dried thyme and dried rosemary

1 tsp salt

1/4 tsp cracked pepper, or to taste

1 pound skinless & boneless chicken thigh fillets or chicken breasts

Salad:

4 cups Romaine lettuce leaves, washed and dried

1 large avocado, pitted, peeled and sliced

8 oz feta cheese

1 cup grape tomatoes, halved

1/4 of a red onion, sliced, optional

1/4 cup diced bacon, trimmed of rind and fat (optional)

Lemon wedges, to serve

Directions:

In a large jug, whisk together the olive oil, lemon juice, water, chopped parsley, garlic, thyme, rosemary, salt, and pepper

Pour half of the marinade into a large, shallow dish and refrigerate the remaining marinade to use as the dressing

Add the chicken to the marinade in the bowl, allow the chicken to marinade for 15- minutes (or up to two hours in the refrigerator if you can)

In the meantime,

Once the chicken is ready, place a skillet or grill over medium-high heat add 1 tbsp of oil in, sear the chicken on both sides until browned and cooked through about 7 minutes per side, depending on thickness, and discard of the marinade

Allow the chicken to rest for 5 minutes, slice and then allow the chicken to cool

Distribute among the containers, and keep in the refrigerator

To Serve: Reheat the chicken in the microwave for 30 seconds to 1 minutes. In a bowl, add the romaine lettuce, avocado, feta cheese, grape tomatoes, red onion and bacon, mix to combine. Arrange the chicken over salad. Drizzle the salad with the Untouched dressing. Serve with lemon wedges and enjoy!

Nutrition Info: Calories:378; Carbs: 6g; Total Fat: 22g; Protein: 31g

Greek-style Braised Pork With Leeks, Greens, And Potatoes

Servings: 4

Cooking Time: 1 Hour 40 Minutes

Ingredients:

1 tablespoon olive oil, plus 2 teaspoons

1¼ pounds boneless pork loin chops, fat cap removed and cut into 1-inch pieces

2 leeks, white and light green parts quartered vertically and thinly sliced

1 bulb fennel, quartered and thinly sliced

1 cup chopped onion

1 teaspoon chopped garlic

2 cups reduced-sodium chicken broth

1 teaspoon fennel seed

1 teaspoon dried oregano

½ teaspoon kosher salt

1 pound baby red potatoes, halved

1 bunch chard, including stems, chopped

2 tablespoons freshly squeezed lemon juice

Directions:

Heat tablespoon of oil in a soup pot or Dutch oven over medium-high heat. When the oil is shimmering, add the pork cubes and brown for about 6 minutes, turning the cubes over after 3 minutes. Remove the pork to a plate.

Add the remaining teaspoons of oil to the same pot and add the leeks, fennel, onion, and garlic. Cook for 3 minutes.

Pour the broth into the pan, scraping up any browned bits on the bottom. Add the fennel seed, oregano, and salt, and add the pork, plus any juices that may have accumulated on the plate. Make sure the pork is submerged in the liquid. Place the potatoes on top, then place the chard on top of the potatoes.

Cover, turn down the heat to low, and simmer for 1½ hours, until the pork is tender. When the pork is done cooking, add the lemon juice. Taste and add more salt if needed. Cool.

Scoop 2 cups of the mixture into each of 4 containers.

STORAGE: Store covered containers in the refrigerator for up to 5 days.

Nutrition Info: Total calories: 3; Total fat: 13g; Saturated fat: 3g; Sodium: 1,607mg; Carbohydrates: 33g; Fiber: 8g; Protein: 34g

Arugula Avocado Salad

Servings: 4

Cooking Time: 15 Minutes

Ingredients:

4 cups packed baby arugula

4 green onions, tops trimmed, chopped

1½ cups shelled fava beans

3 Persian cucumbers, chopped

2 cups grape tomatoes, halved

1 jalapeno pepper, sliced

1 avocado, cored, peeled, and roughly chopped

lemon juice, 1½ lemons

½ cup extra virgin olive oil

salt

pepper

1 garlic clove, finely chopped

2 tablespoons fresh cilantro, finely chopped

2 tablespoons fresh mint, finely chopped

Directions:

Place the lemon-honey vinaigrette Ingredients: in a small bowl and whisk them well.

In a large mixing bowl, add baby arugula, fava beans, green onions, tomatoes, cucumbers, and jalapeno.

Divide the whole salad among four containers.

Before serving, dress the salad with the vinaigrette and toss.

Add the avocado to the salad.

Enjoy!

Nutrition Info: Calories: 229, Total Fat: 11.1 g, Saturated Fat: 2.5 g, Cholesterol: 0 mg, Sodium: 24 mg, Total Carbohydrate: 32.1 g, Dietary Fiber: 12 g, Total Sugars: 10.1 g, Protein: 3 g, Vitamin D: 0 mcg, Calcium: 163 mg, Iron: 3 mg, Potassium: 1166 mg

Quinoa Stuffed Eggplant With Tahini Sauce

Servings: 2

Cooking Time: 30 Minutes

Ingredients:

1 eggplant

2 tbsp olive oil, divided

1 medium shallot, diced, about 1/2 cup

1 cup chopped button mushrooms, about 2 cups whole

5-6 Tuttorosso whole plum tomatoes, chopped

1 tbsp tomato juice from the can

1 tbsp chopped fresh parsley, plus more to garnish

2 garlic cloves, minced

1/2 cup cooked quinoa

1/2 tsp ground cumin

Salt, to taste

Pepper, to taste

1 tbsp tahini

1 tsp lemon juice

1/2 tsp garlic powder

Water to thin

Directions:

Preheat the oven to 425 degrees F

Prepare the eggplant by cutting it in half lengthwise and scoop out some of the flesh

Place it on a baking sheet, drizzle with 1 tbsp of oil, sprinkle with salt

Bake for 20 minutes

In the meantime, add the remaining oil in a large skillet

Once heated, add the shallots and mushrooms, sauté until mushrooms have softened, about 5 minutes Add in the tomatoes, quinoa and spices, cook until the liquid has evaporated

Once the eggplant has cooked, reduce the oven temperature to 350 degrees F

Stuff each half with the tomato-quinoa mixture

Bake for another 10 minutes

Allow to cool completely

Distribute among the containers, store for 2 days

To Serve: Reheat in the microwave for 1-2 minutes or until heated through. Quickly whisk together tahini, lemon, garlic, water and a sprinkle of salt and pepper, drizzle tahini over eggplants and sprinkle with parsley and enjoy.

Nutrition Info: Calories:345; Carbs: 38g; Total Fat: 19g; Protein: 9g

Lasagna

Servings: 8

Cooking Time: 1 Hour 15 Minutes

Ingredients:

Lasagna noodles, oven-ready are the best, easiest, and quickest

⅓ cup flour

2 tablespoons chives, divided and chopped

½ cup white wine

2 tablespoons olive oil

1 ½ tablespoons thyme

1 teaspoon salt

1 ¼ cups shallots, chopped

1 cup boiled water

½ cup Parmigiano-Reggiano cheese

3 cups milk, reduced-fat and divided

1 tablespoon butter

⅓ cup cream cheese, less fat is the best choice

6 cloves of garlic, divided and minced

½ teaspoon ground black pepper, divided

4 ounces dried shiitake mushrooms, sliced

1 ounce dried porcini mushrooms, sliced

8 ounces cremini mushrooms, sliced

Directions:

Keeping your mushrooms separated, drain them all and return them to separate containers.

Bring 1 cup of water to a boil and cook your porcini mushrooms for a half hour.

Preheat your oven to 0 degrees Fahrenheit.

Set a large pan on your stove and turn the burner to medium-high heat.

Add your butter and let it melt.

Combine the olive oil and shallots. Stir the mixture and let it cook for 3 minutes.

Pour half of the pepper, half of the salt, and mushrooms into the pan. Allow the mixture to cook for 6 to minutes.

While stirring, add half of the garlic and thyme. Continue to stir for 1 minute.

Pour the wine and turn your burner temperature to high. Let the mixture boil and watch the liquid evaporate for a couple of minutes to reduce it slightly.

Turn off the burner and remove the pan from heat.

Add the cream cheese and chives. Stir thoroughly.

Set a medium-sized skillet on medium-high heat and add 1 tablespoon of oil. Let the oil come to a simmer.

Add the last of the garlic to the pan and saute for 30 seconds.

Pour in 2 ⅓ cup milk and the liquid from the porcini mushrooms. Stir the mixture and allow it to boil.

In a bowl, combine ¼ cup of milk and the flour. Add this mixture to the heated pan. Stir until the mixture starts to thicken.

Grease a pan and add ½ cup of sauce along with a row of noodles.

Spread half of the mushroom mixture on top of the noodles.

Repeat the process, but make sure you top the lasagna with mushrooms and cheese.

Turn your timer to 45 minutes and set the pan into the oven.

Remember to garnish the lasagna with chives before enjoying!

Nutrition Info: calories: 268, fats: 12.6 grams, carbohydrates: 29 grams, protein: 10 grams.

Tuna With Vegetable Mix

Servings: 4
Cooking Time: 15 Minutes

Ingredients:

¼ cup extra-virgin olive oil, divided

1 tablespoon rice vinegar

1 teaspoon kosher salt, divided

¾ teaspoon Dijon mustard

¾ teaspoon honey

4 ounces baby gold beets, thinly sliced

4 ounces fennel bulb, trimmed and thinly sliced

4 ounces baby turnips, thinly sliced

6 ounces Granny Smith apple, very thinly sliced

2 teaspoons sesame seeds, toasted

6 ounces tuna steaks

½ teaspoon black pepper

1 tablespoon fennel fronds, torn

Directions:

In a large bowl, add 2 tablespoons of oil, ½ a teaspoon of salt, honey, vinegar, and mustard.

Give the mixture a nice mix.

Add fennel, beets, apple, and turnips; mix and toss until everything is evenly coated.

Sprinkle with sesame seeds and toss well.

In a cast-iron skillet, heat 2 tablespoons of oil over high heat.

Carefully season the tuna with ½ a teaspoon of salt and pepper

Place the tuna in the skillet and cook for about 3 minutes total, giving 1½ minutes per side.

Remove the tuna and slice it up.

Place in containers with the vegetable mix.

Serve with the fennel mix, and enjoy!

Nutrition Info: Calories: 443, Total Fat: 17.1 g, Saturated Fat: 2.6 g, Cholesterol: 21 mg, Sodium: 728 mg, Total Carbohydrate: 62.5 g, Dietary Fiber: 12.3 g, Total Sugars: 45 g, Protein: 16.5 g, Vitamin D: 0 mcg, Calcium: 79 mg, Iron: 4 mg, Potassium: 1008 mg

Tuna Bowl With Kale

Servings: 6

Cooking Time: 15 To 20 Minutes

Ingredients:

3 tablespoons extra virgin olive oil

1 ½ teaspoons minced garlic

¼ cup of capers

2 teaspoons sugar

15 ounce can of drained and rinsed great northern beans

1 pound chopped kale with the center ribs removed

½ teaspoon ground black pepper

1 cup chopped onion

2 ½ ounces of drained sliced olives

¼ teaspoon sea salt

¼ teaspoon crushed red pepper

6 ounces of tuna in olive oil, do not drain

Directions:

Place a large pot, like a stockpot, on your stove and turn the burner to high heat.

Fill the pot about 3-quarters of the way full with water and let it come to a boil.

Add the kale and cook for 2 minutes.

Drain the kale and set it aside.

Turn the heat down to medium and place the empty pot back on the burner.

Add the oil and onion. Saute for 3 to 4 minutes.

Combine the garlic into the oil mixture and saute for another minute.

Add the capers, olives, and red pepper.

Cook the ingredients for another minute while stirring.

Pour in the sugar and stir while you toss in the kale. Mix all the ingredients thoroughly and ensure the kale is thoroughly coated.

Cover the pot and set the timer for 8 minutes.

Turn off the heat and add in the tuna, pepper, beans, salt, and any other herbs that will make this one of the best Mediterranean dishes you've ever made.

Nutrition Info: calories: 265, fats: 12 grams, carbohydrates: 26 grams, protein: 16 grams.

Tomato Soup

Servings: 8

Cooking Time: 30 Minutes

Ingredients:

4 tablespoons olive oil

2 medium yellow onions, thinly sliced

1 teaspoon salt (extra for taste if needed)

2 teaspoons curry powder

1 teaspoon red curry powder

1 teaspoon ground coriander

1 teaspoon ground cumin

¼-½ teaspoon red pepper flakes

1 15-ounce can diced tomatoes, undrained

1 28-ounce can diced or plum tomatoes, undrained

5½ cups water (vegetable broth or chicken broth also usable)

1 14-ounce can coconut milk

optional add-ins: cooked brown rice, lemon wedges, fresh thyme, etc.

Directions:

Heat oil in a medium-sized pot over medium heat.

Add onions and salt and cook for about 10-1minutes until browned.

Stir in curry powder, coriander, red pepper flakes, cumin, and cook for seconds, being sure to keep stirring well.

Add tomatoes and water (or broth if you prefer).

Simmer the mixture for 1minutes.

Take an immersion blender and puree the mixture until a soupy consistency is achieved.

Enjoy as it is, or add some extra add-ins for a more flavorful experience.

Nutrition Info: Calories: 217, Total Fat: 19.3 g, Saturated Fat: 11.5 g, Cholesterol: 0 mg, Sodium: 40 mg, Total Carbohydrate: 12.1 g, Dietary Fiber: 3.g, Total Sugars: 7.1 g, Protein: 3 g, Vitamin D: 0 mcg, Calcium: 58 mg, Iron: 2 mg, Potassium: 570 mg

Cheese Onion Soup

Servings: 4

Cooking Time: 25 Minutes

Ingredients:

2 large onions, finely sliced

2 cups vegetable stock

1 teaspoon brown sugar

1 cup red wine

1 measure of brandy

1 teaspoon herbs de Provence

4 slices stale bread

4 ounces grated strong cheese

1-ounce grated parmesan

1 tablespoon plain flour

2 tablespoons olive oil

1-ounce butter

salt

pepper

Directions:

Heat oil and butter in a pan over medium-high heat.

Add onions and brown sugar.

Cook until the onions are golden brown.

Pour brandy and flambé, making sure to keep stirring until the flames are out.

Add plain flour and herbs de Provence and keep stirring well.

Slowly add the stock and red wine.

Season well and simmer for 20 minutes, making sure to add water if the soup becomes too thick.

Ladle the soup into jars.

Before serving, place rounds of stale bread on top.

Add strong cheese.

Garnish with some parmesan.

Place the bowls under a hot grill or in an oven until the cheese has melted.

Nutrition Info: Calories: 403, Total Fat: 22.4 g, Saturated Fat: 10.9 g, Cholesterol: 41 mg, Sodium: 886 mg, Total Carbohydrate: 24.9 g, Dietary Fiber: 3.6 g, Total Sugars: 7 g, Protein: 16.2 g, Vitamin D: 4 mcg, Calcium: 371 mg, Iron: 1 mg, Potassium: 242 mg

SAUCES AND DRESSINGS RECIPES

Bulgur Pilaf With Almonds

Servings: 4

Cooking Time: 20 Minutes

Ingredients:

⅔ cup uncooked bulgur

1⅓ cups water

¼ cup sliced almonds

1 cup small diced red bell pepper

⅓ cup chopped fresh cilantro

1 tablespoon olive oil

¼ teaspoon salt

Directions:

Place the bulgur and water in a saucepan and bring the water to a boil. Once the water is at a boil, cover the pot with a lid and turn off the heat. Let the covered pot stand for 20 minutes. Transfer the cooked bulgur to a large mixing bowl and add the almonds, peppers, cilantro, oil, and salt. Stir to combine. Place about 1 cup of bulgur in each of 4 containers.

STORAGE: Store covered containers in the refrigerator for up to 5 days. Bulgur can be either reheated or eaten at room temperature.

Nutrition Info: Total calories: 17 Total fat: 7g; Saturated fat: 1g; Sodium: 152mg; Carbohydrates: 25g; Fiber: 6g; Protein: 4g

Garlic Yogurt Sauce

Servings: 1 Cup

Cooking Time: 5 Minutes

Ingredients:

1 cup low-fat (2%) plain Greek yogurt

½ teaspoon garlic powder

1 tablespoon freshly squeezed lemon juice

1 tablespoon olive oil

¼ teaspoon kosher salt

Directions:

Mix all the ingredients in a medium bowl until well combined.

Spoon the yogurt sauce into a container and refrigerate.

STORAGE: Store the covered container in the refrigerator for up to 7 days.

Nutrition Info: Per Serving (¼ cup): Total calories: 75; Total fat: 5g; Saturated fat: 1g; Sodium: 173mg; Carbohydrates: 3g; Fiber: 0g; Protein: 6g.

DESSERTS RECIPES

Cherry Brownies With Walnuts

Servings: 9

Cooking Time: 25 To 30 Minutes

Ingredients:

9 fresh cherries that are stemmed and pitted or 9 frozen cherries

½ cup sugar or sweetener substitute

¼ cup extra virgin olive oil

1 teaspoon vanilla extract

¼ teaspoon sea salt

½ cup whole-wheat pastry flour

¼ teaspoon baking powder

⅓ cup walnuts, chopped

2 eggs

½ cup plain Greek yogurt

⅓ cup cocoa powder, unsweetened

Directions:

Make sure one of the metal racks in your oven is set in the middle.

Turn the temperature on your oven to 375 degrees Fahrenheit.

Using cooking spray, grease a 9-inch square pan.

Take a large bowl and add the oil and sugar or sweetener substitute. Whisk the ingredients well.

Add the eggs and use a mixer to beat the ingredients together.

Pour in the yogurt and continue to beat the mixture until it is smooth.

Take a medium bowl and combine the cocoa powder, flour, sea salt, and baking powder by whisking them together.

Combine the powdered ingredients into the wet ingredients and use your electronic mixer to incorporate the ingredients together thoroughly.

Add in the walnuts and stir.

Pour the mixture into the pan.

Sprinkle the cherries on top and push them into the batter. You can use any design, but it is best to make three rows and three columns with the cherries. This ensures that each piece of the brownie will have one cherry.

Put the batter into the oven and turn your timer to 20 minutes.

Check that the brownies are done using the toothpick test before removing them from the oven. Push the toothpick into the middle of the brownies and once it comes out clean, remove the brownies.

Let the brownies cool for 5 to 10 minutes before cutting and serving.

Nutrition Info: calories: 225, fats: 10 grams, carbohydrates: 30 grams, protein: 5 grams.

Fruit Dip

Servings: 10
Cooking Time: 10 To 15 Minutes

Ingredients:
¼ cup coconut milk, full-fat is best
¼ cup vanilla yogurt
⅓ cup marshmallow creme
1 cup cream cheese, set at room temperature
2 tablespoons maraschino cherry juice

Directions:
In a large bowl, add the coconut milk, vanilla yogurt, marshmallow creme, cream cheese, and cherry juice.
Using an electric mixer, set to low speed and blend the ingredients together until the fruit dip is smooth.
Serve the dip with some of your favorite fruits and enjoy!

Nutrition Info: calories: 110, fats: 11 grams, carbohydrates: 3 grams, protein: 3 grams.

A Lemony Treat

Servings: 4

Cooking Time: 30 Minutes

Ingredients:

1 lemon, medium in size

1 ½ teaspoons cornstarch

1 cup Greek yogurt, plain is best

Fresh fruit

¼ cup cold water

⅔ cup heavy whipped cream

3 tablespoons honey

Optional: mint leaves

Directions:

Take a large glass bowl and your metal, electric mixer and set them in the refrigerator so they can chill.

In a separate bowl, add the yogurt and set that in the fridge.

Zest the lemon into a medium bowl that is microwavable.

Cut the lemon in half and then squeeze 1 tablespoon of lemon juice into the bowl.

Combine the cornstarch and water. Mix the ingredients thoroughly.

Pour in the honey and whisk the ingredients together.

Put the mixture into the microwave for 1 minute on high.

Once the microwave stops, remove the mixture and stir.

Set it back into the microwave for 15 to 30 seconds or until the mixture starts to bubble and thicken.

Take the bowl of yogurt from the fridge and pour in the warm mixture while whisking.

Put the yogurt mixture back into the fridge.

Take the large bowl and beaters out of the fridge.

Put your electronic mixer together and pour the whipped cream into the chilled bowl.

Beat the cream until soft peaks start to form. This can take up to 3 minutes, depending on how fresh your cream is.

Remove the yogurt from the fridge.

Fold the yogurt into the cream using a rubber spatula. Remember to lift and turn the mixture so it doesn't deflate.

Place back into the fridge until you are serving the dessert or for 15 minutes. The dessert should not be in the fridge for longer than 1 hour.

When you serve the lemony goodness, you will spoon it into four dessert dishes and drizzle with extra honey or even melt some chocolate to drizzle on top.

Add a little fresh mint and enjoy!

Nutrition Info: calories: 241, fats: 16 grams, carbohydrates: 21 grams, protein: 7 grams.

Melon With Ginger

Servings: 4

Cooking Time: 10 To 15 Minutes

Ingredients:

½ cantaloupe, cut into 1-inch chunks

2 cups of watermelon, cut into 1-inch chunks

2 cups honeydew melon, cut into 1-inch chunks

2 tablespoons of raw honey

Ginger, 2 inches in size, peeled, grated, and preserve the juice

Directions:

In a large bowl, combine your cantaloupe, honeydew melon, and watermelon. Gently mix the ingredients.

Combine the ginger juice and stir.

Drizzle on the honey, serve, and enjoy! You can also chill the mixture for up to an hour before serving.

Nutrition Info: calories: 91, fats: 0 grams, carbohydrates: 23 grams, protein: 1 gram.

Almond Shortbread Cookies

Servings: 16

Cooking Time: 25 Minutes

Ingredients:

½ cup coconut oil

1 teaspoon vanilla extract

2 egg yolks

1 tablespoon brandy

1 cup powdered sugar

1 cup finely ground almonds

3 ½ cups cake flour

½ cup almond butter

1 tablespoon water or rose flower water

Directions:

In a large bowl, combine the coconut oil, powdered sugar, and butter. If the butter is not soft, you want to wait until it softens up. Use an electric mixer to beat the ingredients together at high speed.

In a small bowl, add the egg yolks, brandy, water, and vanilla extract. Whisk well.

Fold the egg yolk mixture into the large bowl.

Add the flour and almonds. Fold and mix with a wooden spoon.

Place the mixture into the fridge for at least 1 hour and 30 minutes.

Preheat your oven to 325 degrees Fahrenheit.

Take the mixture, which now looks like dough, and divide it into 1-inch balls.

With a piece of parchment paper on a baking sheet, arrange the cookies and flatten them with a fork or your fingers.

Place the cookies in the oven for 13 minutes, but watch them so they don't burn.

Transfer the cookies onto a rack to cool for a couple of minutes before enjoying!

Nutrition Info: calories: 250, fats: 14 grams, carbohydrates: 30 grams, protein: 3 grams.

Peaches With Blue Cheese Cream

Servings: 4

Cooking Time: 20 Hours 10 Minutes

Ingredients:

4 peaches

1 cinnamon stick

4 ounces sliced blue cheese

⅓ cup orange juice, freshly squeezed is best

3 whole cloves

1 teaspoon of orange zest, taken from the orange peel

¼ teaspoon cardamom pods

⅔ cup red wine

2 tablespoons honey, raw or your preferred variety

1 vanilla bean

1 teaspoon allspice berries

4 tablespoons dried cherries

Directions:

Set a saucepan on top of your stove range and add the cinnamon stick, cloves, orange juice, cardamom, vanilla, allspice, red wine, and orange zest. Whisk the ingredients well.

Add your peaches to the mixture and poach them for hours or until they become soft.

Take a spoon to remove the peaches and boil the rest of the liquid to make the syrup. You want the liquid to reduce itself by at least half.

While the liquid is boiling, combine the dried cherries, blue cheese, and honey into a bowl.

Once your peaches are cooled, slice them into halves.

Top each peach with the blue cheese mixture and then drizzle the liquid onto the top.

Serve and enjoy!

Nutrition Info: calories: 211, fats: 24 grams, carbohydrates: 15 grams, protein: 6 grams.

Mediterranean Blackberry Ice Cream

Servings: 6

Cooking Time: 15 Minutes

Ingredients:

3 egg yolks

1 container of Greek yogurt

1 pound mashed blackberries

½ teaspoon vanilla essence

1 teaspoon arrowroot powder

¼ teaspoon ground cloves

5 ounces sugar or sweetener substitute

1 pound heavy cream

Directions:

In a small bowl, add the arrowroot powder and egg yolks. Whisk or beat them with an electronic mixture until they are well combined.

Set a saucepan on top of your stove and turn your heat to medium.

Add the heavy cream and bring it to a boil.

Turn off the heat and add the egg mixture into the cream through folding.

Turn the heat back on to medium and pour in the sugar. Cook the mixture for 10 minutes or until it starts to thicken.

Remove the mixture from heat and place it in the fridge so it can completely cool. This should take about one hour.

Once the mixture is cooled, add in the Greek yogurt, ground cloves, blackberries, and vanilla by folding in the ingredients.

Transfer the ice cream into a container and place it in the freezer for at least two hours.

Serve and enjoy!

Nutrition Info: calories: 402, fats: 20 grams, carbohydrates: 52 grams, protein: 8 grams.

Stuffed Figs

Servings: 6

Cooking Time: 20 Minutes

Ingredients:

10 halved fresh figs

20 chopped almonds

4 ounces goat cheese, divided

2 tablespoons of raw honey

Directions:

Turn your oven to broiler mode and set it to a high temperature.

Place your figs, cut side up, on a baking sheet. If you like to place a piece of parchment paper on top you can do this, but it is not necessary.

Sprinkle each fig with half of the goat cheese.

Add a tablespoon of chopped almonds to each fig.

Broil the figs for 3 to 4 minutes.

Take them out of the oven and let them cool for 5 to 7 minutes.

Sprinkle with the remaining goat cheese and honey.

Nutrition Info: calories: 209, fats: 9 grams, carbohydrates: 26 grams, protein: grams.

Chia Pudding With Strawberries

Servings: 4

Cooking Time: 4 Hours 5 Minutes

Ingredients:

2 cups unsweetened almond milk

1 tablespoon vanilla extract

2 tablespoons raw honey

¼ cup chia seeds

2 cups fresh and sliced strawberries

Directions:

In a medium bowl, combine the honey, chia seeds, vanilla, and unsweetened almond milk. Mix well.

Set the mixture in the refrigerator for at least 4 hours.

When you serve the pudding, top it with strawberries. You can even create a design in a glass serving bowl or dessert dish by adding a little pudding on the bottom, a few strawberries, top the strawberries with some more pudding, and then top the dish with a few strawberries.

Nutrition Info: calories: 108, fats: grams, carbohydrates: 17 grams, protein: 3 grams.

SIDES & APPETIZERS RECIPES

Chicken Bacon Pasta

Servings: 4
Cooking Time: 35 Minutes

Ingredients:

8 ounces linguine pasta

3 slices of bacon

1 pound boneless chicken breast, cooked and diced

salt

2 ounce can diced tomatoes, undrained

¼ teaspoon dried rosemary

1/3 cup crumbled feta cheese, plus extra for topping

2/3 cup pitted black olives

1 6-ounce can artichoke hearts

Directions:

Fill a large pot with salted water and bring to a boil.

Add linguine and cook for 8-10 minutes until al dente.

Cook bacon until brown, and then crumble.

Season chicken with salt.

Place chicken and bacon into a large skillet.

Add tomatoes and rosemary and simmer the mixture for about 20 minutes.

Stir in feta cheese, artichoke hearts, and olives, and cook until thoroughly heated.

Toss the freshly cooked pasta with chicken mixture and cool.

Spread over the containers.

Before eating, garnish with extra feta if your heart desires!

Nutrition Info: Calories: 755, Total Fat: 22.5 g, Saturated Fat: 6.5 g, Cholesterol: 128 mg, Sodium: 852 mg, Total Carbohydrate: 75.4 g, Dietary Fiber: 7.3 g, Total Sugars: 3.4 g, Protein: 55.6 g, Vitamin D: 0 mcg, Calcium: 162 mg, Iron: 7 mg, Potassium: 524 mg

Creamy Garlic Shrimp Pasta

Servings: 4
Cooking Time: 15 Minutes

Ingredients:

6 ounces whole-wheat spaghetti, your favorite

12 ounces raw shrimp, peeled, deveined, and cut into 1-inch pieces

1 bunch asparagus, trimmed and thinly sliced

1 large bell pepper, thinly sliced

3 cloves garlic, chopped

1¼ teaspoon kosher salt

1½ cups non-fat plain yogurt

¼ cup flat-leaf parsley, chopped

3 tablespoons lemon juice

1 tablespoon extra virgin olive oil

½ teaspoon fresh ground black pepper

¼ cup toasted pine nuts

Directions:

Bring water to a boil in a large pot.

Add spaghetti and cook for about minutes less than called for by the package instructions.

Add shrimp, bell pepper, asparagus and cook for about 2-4 minutes until the shrimp are tender.

Drain the pasta.

In a large bowl, mash the garlic until paste forms.

Whisk yogurt, parsley, oil, pepper, and lemon juice into the garlic paste.

Add pasta mixture and toss well.

Cool and spread over the containers.

Sprinkle with pine nuts.

Enjoy!

Nutrition Info: Calories: 504, Total Fat: 15.4 g, Saturated Fat: 4.9 g, Cholesterol: 199 mg, Sodium: 2052 mg, Total Carbohydrate: 42.2 g, Dietary Fiber: 3.5 g, Total Sugars: 26.6 g, Protein: 43.2 g, Vitamin D: 0 mcg, Calcium: 723 mg, Iron: 3 mg, Potassium: 3 mg

Mushroom Fettuccine

Servings: 5

Cooking Time: 15 Minutes

Ingredients:

12 ounces whole-wheat fettuccine (or any other)

1 tablespoon extra virgin olive oil

4 cups mixed mushrooms, such as oyster, cremini, etc., sliced

4 cups broccoli, divided

1 tablespoon minced garlic

½ cup dry sherry

2 cups low-fat milk

2 tablespoons all-purpose flour

½ teaspoon salt

½ teaspoon freshly ground pepper

1 cup finely shredded Asiago cheese, plus some for topping

Directions:

Cook pasta in a large pot of boiling water for about 8- minutes.

Drain pasta and set it to the side.

Add oil to large skillet and heat over medium heat.

Add mushrooms and broccoli, and cook for about 8-10 minutes until the mushrooms have released the liquid.

Add garlic and cook for about 1 minute until fragrant.

Add sherry, making sure to scrape up any brown bits.

Bring the mix to a boil and cook for about 1 minute until evaporated.

In a separate bowl, whisk flour and milk.

Add the mix to your skillet, and season with salt and pepper.

Cook well for about 2 minutes until the sauce begins to bubble and is thickened.

Stir in Asiago cheese until it has fully melted.

Add the sauce to your pasta and give it a gentle toss.

Spread over the containers. Serve with extra cheese.

Nutrition Info: Calories: 503, Total Fat: 19.6 g, Saturated Fat: 6.3 g, Cholesterol: 25 mg, Sodium: 1136 mg, Total Carbohydrate: 57.5 g, Dietary Fiber: 12.4 g, Total Sugars: 6.4 g, Protein: 24.5 g, Vitamin D: 51 mcg, Calcium: 419 mg, Iron: 5 mg, Potassium: 390 mg

Lemon Garlic Sardine Fettuccine

Servings: 4

Cooking Time: 15 Minutes

Ingredients:

8 ounces whole-wheat fettuccine

4 tablespoons extra-virgin olive oil, divided

4 cloves garlic, minced

1 cup fresh breadcrumbs

¼ cup lemon juice

1 teaspoon freshly ground pepper

½ teaspoon of salt

2 4-ounce cans boneless and skinless sardines, dipped in tomato sauce

½ cup fresh parsley, chopped

¼ cup finely shredded parmesan cheese

Directions:

Fill a large pot with water and bring to a boil.

Cook pasta according to package instructions until tender (about 10 minutes).

In a small skillet, heat 2 tablespoons of oil over medium heat.

Add garlic and cook for about 20 seconds, until sizzling and fragrant.

Transfer the garlic to a large bowl.

Add the remaining 2 tablespoons of oil to skillet and heat over medium heat.

Add breadcrumbs and cook for 5-6 minutes until golden and crispy.

Whisk lemon juice, salt, and pepper into the garlic bowl.

Add pasta to the garlic bowl, along with garlic, sardines, parmesan, and parsley; give it a gentle stir.

Cool and spread over the containers.

Before eating, sprinkle with breadcrumbs.

Enjoy!

Nutrition Info: Calories: 633, Total Fat: 27.7 g, Saturated Fat: 6.4 g, Cholesterol: 40 mg, Sodium: 771 mg, Total Carbohydrate: 55.9 g, Dietary Fiber: 7.7 g, Total Sugars: 2.1 g, Protein: 38.6 g, Vitamin D: 0 mcg, Calcium: 274 mg, Iron: 7 mg, Potassium: mg

Spinach Almond Stir-fry

Servings: 2

Cooking Time: 10 Minutes

Ingredients:

2 ounces spinach

1 tablespoon coconut oil

3 tablespoons almond, slices

sea salt or plain salt

freshly ground black pepper

Directions:

Start by heating a skillet with coconut oil; add spinach and let it cook.

Then, add salt and pepper as the spinach is cooking.

Finally, add in the almond slices.

Serve warm.

Nutrition Info: Calories: 117, Total Fat: 11.4 g, Saturated Fat: 6.2 g, Cholesterol: 0 mg, Sodium: 23 mg, Total Carbohydrate: 2.9 g, Dietary Fiber: 1.7 g, Total Sugars: 0.g, Protein: 2.7 g, Vitamin D: 0 mcg, Calcium: 52 mg, Iron: 1 mg, Potassium: 224 mg

Bbq Carrots

Servings: 8
Cooking Time: 30 Minutes

Ingredients:

2 pounds baby carrots (organic)
1 tablespoon olive oil
1 tablespoon garlic powder
1 tablespoon onion powder
sea salt or plain salt
freshly ground black pepper

Directions:

Mix all the Ingredients: in a plastic bag so that the carrots are well coated with the mixture.

Then, on the BBQ grill place a piece of aluminum foil and spread the carrots in a single layer.

Finally, grill for 30 minutes or until tender.

Serve warm.

Nutrition Info: Calories: 388, Total Fat: 1.9 g, Saturated Fat: 0.3 g, Cholesterol: 0 mg, Sodium: 89 mg, Total Carbohydrate: 10.8 g, Dietary Fiber: 3.4 g, Total Sugars: 6 g, Protein: 1 g, Vitamin D: 0 mcg, Calcium: 40 mg, Iron: 1 mg, Potassium: 288 mg

GREAT MEDITERRANEAN DIET RECIPES

Sicilian style fish stew

Preparation time: 10 minutes

Cooking time: 35 minutes

Servings: 6

Ingredients:

Olive oil

Two chopped celery ribs chopped yellow onion

Salt to taste

Four minced garlic cloves tbsp toasted pine nuts

Black pepper to taste

½ tsp dried thyme

¾ cup dry white wine

One pinch of red pepper flakes

28 oz plum tomatoes

Tomato juice

¼ cup golden raisins cups vegetable broth

2 tbsp capers

½ cup chopped parsley leaves

2 lb sliced skinless bass fillet

Italian bread for serving

Directions :

Sauté onions and celery, black pepper, and salt in a Dutch oven over medium flame with constant stirring for four minutes.

Add flakes, thyme, and garlic, and cook for one minute.

Mix tomato juice and white wine and let it simmer.

When the liquid is concentrated to half, add capers, tomatoes, raisins, and stock.

Cook for 20 more minutes.

Rub fish with pepper and salt and add in cooking solution and mix well. Let it simmer for five minutes.

Remove from the flame and let it cool for five minutes while the oven is covered.

Sprinkle parsley and pine nuts and serve.

Nutrition Info: Calories: 320 kcal Fat:11.6 g Protein: 31.2 g Carbs: 19.8 g Fiber: 2.8 g

Chicken souvlaki

Preparation time: 45 minutes

Cooking time: 40 minutes

Servings: 4

Ingredients:

Margination

12 boneless chicken thighs

4 tbsp olive oil tsp dried mint tsp dried oregano

1 tsp ground cumin

1 tsp sweet paprika crushed garlic cloves

1 tsp coriander

½ tsp ground cinnamon

1 tbsp lemon juice

Zest of one lemon

Wedges cut slices of one lemon slices

Pitta wraps

250 g white bread flour tsp caster sugar

7 g dried yeast tsp olive oil

Tzatziki sauce

crushed garlic clove

½ chopped cucumber

small bunch of chopped mint leaves

200 g Greek yogurt

1 tbsp lemon juice

To serve

Four chopped tomatoes One lettuce
One sliced red onion

Directions : In a large mixing bowl, add chicken and black pepper, salt, and all the ingredients mentioned in the marination list. Toss to coat well. Leave it overnight for better results in the refrigerator.

Whisk flour, sugar, salt, and yeast in a bowl. Pour 2 tsp oil and warm water about 150 ml and mix to form a dough. Knead the dough for ten minutes.

Cover the bowl and set aside for 60 minutes.

Make four portions of the raised dough, roll them into circles, and set aside 20 more minutes. The dough for pita bread is ready.

In a bowl, mix all the ingredients of the Tzatziki sauce and set aside. The Tzatziki sauce is ready.

Thread chicken pieces on skewers separately, place the skewers over the top of roasting tin, place overheated grill, and cook the chicken for 20 minutes while brushing with oil. When chicken is done, set aside.

Brush the flattened pita bread with oil and place in a heated pan. Cook for three minutes, and when it turned golden from the underside, then flip and cook the other side for three more minutes. When the bread is fully cooked, cover it and keep it warm until further use.

Make kebabs out of grilled chicken and place in pita bread followed by tomato, onion, lettuce, lemon slices, and drizzle Tzatziki sauce and serve.

Nutrition Info: Calories: 707 kcal Fat: 34 g Protein: 46 g Carbs: 52 g Fiber: 4 g

Grilled swordfish

Preparation time: 15 minutes

Cooking time: 8 minutes

Servings: 4

Ingredients:

Ten garlic cloves

2 tbsp lemon juice

1/3 cup olive oil 2 tsp coriander

1 tsp Spanish paprika

¾ tsp cumin

¾ tsp salt

Four swordfish steaks

½ tsp black pepper

Crushed red pepper to taste

Directions : Blend olive oil, pepper, garlic, salt, and lemon juice in a blender to obtain a smooth mixture. Coat swordfish with the garlic blended mixture and keep it aside for 15 minutes. Heat grill on high flame. Place fish and cook for five minutes from each side.

Sprinkle lemon juice and flakes and serve.

Nutrition Info: Calories: 398 kcal Fat: 30.7 g Protein: 28.4 g Carbs: 3.1 g Fiber: 0.6 g

Greek shrimp with tomatoes and feta

Preparation time: 10 minutes

Cooking time: 40 minutes

Servings: 4

Ingredients:

4 tbsp olive oil

3/4 cup chopped shallots

Four chopped garlic cloves

28 oz diced tomatoes 1 tsp salt

1/4 tsp pepper 2 tsp cumin

1/2 tsp crushed pepper flakes

1 tbsp honey

1.5 lb shrimp

6 oz feta cheese

3/4 tsp dried oregano 2 tbsp chopped mint

Directions :

Cook garlic and shallots in heated oil in a skillet over low flame for eight minutes.

Stir in salt, cumin, honey, tomatoes, tomato juices, flakes, and pepper.

Let the sauce boil and cook for 20 minutes with occasional stirring.

Remove from flame and add shrimps in the sauce. Sprinkle feta cheese and oregano.

Bake in a preheated oven at 400 degrees for 15 minutes. Shift the shrimp pan to broil and broil for two minutes. Garnish with mint and serve.

Nutrition Info: Calories: 431 kcal Fat: 25 g Protein: 32 g Carbs: 21 g Fiber: 5 g

Salmon kabobs

Preparation time: 10 minutes

Cooking time: 8 minutes

Servings: 6

Ingredients:

1.5 lb sliced Salmon fillet

One sliced red onion

One sliced zucchini

Kosher salt to taste

Black pepper to taste

Marinade

1/3 cup Olive Oil

Zest of one lemon 2 tbsp lemon juice minced garlic cloves

1 tsp chili pepper 2 tsp dry oregano

2 tsp chopped thyme leaves

1 tsp cumin

½ tsp coriander

Directions :

Mix all the ingredients of margination in a bowl.

In another bowl, add pepper, onions, salt, salmon, and zucchini and mix well.

Add marinade and mix well. Set aside for 20 minutes.

Thread onions, salmon, and zucchini in skewers.

Place skewers overheated grill, cover them, and grill for eight minutes.

When salmons are ready, serve and enjoy it.

Nutrition Info: Calories: 267 kcal Fat: 11 g Protein: 35 g Carbs: 7 g Fiber: 3 g

Greek chicken and potatoes

Preparation time: 10 minutes

Cooking time: 50 minutes

Servings: 4

Ingredients:

4 lb chicken thighs 2 tbsp oregano

1 tbsp salt

1 tsp black pepper

2/3 cup chicken stock

One pinch of cayenne pepper

1 tsp rosemary

½ cup lemon juice

Six minced garlic cloves

½ cup olive oil

Three sliced russet potatoes

1 tbsp chopped oregano

Directions :

Add lemon juice, oregano, oil, cayenne pepper, salt, garlic, rosemary, black pepper potatoes, and chicken in a bowl. Mix them to coat everything well.

Place chicken in a roasting tray.

Spread potato pieces, 2/3 cup of stock, and marinade over chicken pieces.

Bake in a preheated oven at 425 degrees for 20 minutes.

Change the sides of the chicken and bake for 20 more minutes. Bake until chicken is done and shift chicken in serving dish. Mix potatoes with remaining juice and broil for three minutes. Shift the potatoes in the serving dish beside the chicken. Concentrate chicken stock left in a roasting tray on the stove over medium flame.

Nutrition Info: Calories: 138 kcal Fat: 74.5 g Protein: 80.4 g Carbs: 34.4 g Fiber: 3 g

Italian style baked fish

Preparation time: 5 minutes

Cooking time: 30 minutes

Servings: 6

Ingredients:

1/3 cup olive oil

Two diced tomatoes 1.5 chopped red onion

Ten chopped garlic cloves

1 tsp Spanish paprika 2 tsp coriander

1 tsp cumin

1.5 tbsp capers

½ tsp cayenne pepper

Salt to taste

1/3 cup raisins

1 tbsp of lemon juice

Black pepper to taste

Parsley for garnishing

Zest of one lemon

1.5 lb white fish fillet

Mint for garnishing

Directions :

Cook onions in heated olive oil in a saucepan for three minutes.
Stir in tomatoes, salt, capers, garlic, raisins, and spices and let
them boil.

Reduce the flame to low and simmer for 15 minutes.

Rub fish with pepper and salt and set aside.

Transfer half of the cooked tomato mixture to the baking pan, followed by fish, lemon juice, zest, and leftover tomato mixture.

Bake in a preheated oven at 400 degrees for 18 minutes.

Sprinkle mint and parsley and serve.

Nutrition Info: Calories: 308 kcal Fat: 17.4 g Protein: 27 g Carbs: 13.3 g Fiber: 2 g

Tzatziki sauce and dip

Preparation time: 10 minutes

Cooking time: 0 minute

Servings: 4

Ingredients:

½ halved cucumber

3/4 cup Yogurt

Two minced garlic cloves2 tbsp red wine vinegar

1 tbsp minced dill

One pinch of kosher salt

One pinch of black pepper

Directions : Place dried shredded cucumber in a bowl.

Mix garlic, vinegar, salt, yogurt, dill, and pepper in cucumber
and mix well.

Cover the bowl and place it in the refrigerator. The Tzatziki
sauce is ready.

Can store up to three days.

Nutrition Info: Calories: 30 kcal Fat: 1 g Protein: 4 g Carbs: 3
g Fiber: 1 g

Pesto and garlic shrimp bruschetta

Preparation time: 10 minutes

Cooking time: 15 minutes

Servings: 12

Ingredients:

8 oz shrimp

Black pepper to taste

2 tbsp butter

4 tbsp olive oil

20 basil leaves One bread

Four minced garlic cloves3 oz pesto

2 oz capers3 oz sun-dried tomatoes

1 oz feta cheese

kosher salt to taste

Glaze Balsamic for garnishing

Directions : Sprinkle salt and pepper over shrimps in a bowl.
Set aside for ten minutes.

Add olive oil and butter of about 2 tbsp each in the pan and cook for 2 minutes over medium flame.

Stir in garlic and sauté for one more minute.

Mix shrimps and cook for four minutes.

Remove from flame and let it set.

Slice the bread and place in a baking tray and drizzle oil and toast in the oven for five minutes.

Spread pesto sauce over each bread slice followed by sun-dried tomatoes, shrimp, caper, cheese, basil, and balsamic glaze and serve.

Nutrition Info: Calories: 168 kcal Fat: 7 g Protein: 5 g Carbs: 19 g Fiber: 1 g

Cucumber and tomato salad

Preparation time: 10 minutes

Cooking time: 0 minute

Servings: 4

Ingredients:

One sliced English cucumber

½ sliced red onion

Three diced tomatoes

2 tbsp olive oil

Salt to taste

1 tbsp red wine vinegar

Black pepper to taste

Directions : In a large mixing bowl, mix all the ingredients and place in the refrigerator for 20 minutes.

Serve and enjoy it.

Nutrition Info: Calories: 104 kcal Fat: 8 g Protein: 2 g Carbs: 7 g Fiber: 2 g

Citrus avocado dip

Preparation time: 15 minutes

Cooking time: 0 minute

Servings: 8

Ingredients:

Two diced oranges

½ cup chopped onions

½ cup chopped mint

½ cup chopped cilantro

Olive oil as required

Two sliced avocados

½ cup chopped walnuts

Black pepper to taste

Cayenne as required

Salt to taste

1 tbsp of lime juice

¾ tsp sumac

1.75 oz shredded feta cheese

Directions : In a bowl, combine all the ingredients and mix well.

Serve and enjoy it.

Nutrition Info: Calories: 147 kcal Fat: 10.3 g Protein: 2.8 g Carbs: 14.6 g Fiber: 2.1 g

Roasted tomatoes with thyme and feta

Preparation time: 5 minutes

Cooking time: 20 minutes

Servings: 4

Ingredients:

½ tsp dried thyme

16 oz cherry tomatoes

Black pepper to taste

3 tbsp olive oil

Salt to taste

6 tbsp feta cheese

Directions : In a baking tray, put tomatoes.

Pour olive oil and drizzle pepper, thyme leaves, and salt over tomatoes and mix well.

Bake in a preheated oven at 450 degrees for 15 minutes.

Drizzle cheese and broil for five minutes and serve when the cheese melts.

Nutrition Info: Calories: 195 kcal Fat: 7.3 g Protein: 2 g Carbs: 3.1 g Fiber: 1.1 g

Greek salad

Preparation time: 20 minutes

Cooking time: 0 minute

Servings: 5

Ingredients:

Dressing

6 tbsp olive oil

¾ tsp honey

1 tbsp red wine vinegar

1/5 tbsp lemon juice

1.5 tsp minced garlic

1 tsp oregano

1.5 tbsp minced parsley

Salt to taste

Salad

Four diced tomatoes

½ chopped onion

One chopped English cucumber

One chopped green bell pepper

4 oz feta cheese

¾ cup sliced Kalamata olives

One chopped avocado

Directions :

Whisk all the ingredients mentioned in the dressing list in a large mixing bowl. Set aside. In another bowl, add all the ingredients of the salad and toss well.

Pour the dressing, toss well and serve.

Nutrition Info: Calories: 248 kcal Fat: 24 g Protein: 3 g Carbs: 4 g Fiber: 1 g

Creamiest Hummus

Preparation time: 5 minutes

Cooking time: 0 minute

Servings: 10

Ingredients:

400 g chickpeas

½ tsp salt

8 tbsp tahini

10 tbsp liquid from chickpeas can

2 tbsp lemon juice

1 tbsp olive oil

Directions :

In a food processor, blend chickpeas, lemon juice, tahini, salt, and aquafaba to get smooth hummus.

Transfer the blended hummus to the bowl. Pour olive oil in the center of the hummus and serve.

Nutrition Info: Calories: 100 kcal Fat: 7 g Protein: 3 g Carbs: 5 g Fiber: 3 g

Roasted cauliflower with lemon and cumin

Preparation time: 15 minutes

Cooking time: 25 minutes

Servings: 4

Ingredients:

11 oz cauliflower

1 tbsp of lemon juice

1/3 cup olive oil

Salt to taste

Zest of one lemon

1 tbsp ground sumac

1 tbsp ground cumin

1 tsp garlic powder

Black pepper to taste

Directions :

Mix all the ingredients in a large mixing bowl.

Transfer the cauliflower to a baking tray and bake in a preheated oven at 425 degrees for 25 minutes.

Serve and enjoy it.

Nutrition Info: Calories: 213 kcal Fat: 18 g Protein: 3 g Carbs: 10 g Fiber: 3 g

Tabbouleh salad

Preparation time: 20 minutes

Cooking time: 0 minute

Servings: 6

Ingredients:

½ cup bulgur wheat

One chopped English cucumber

Four chopped tomatoes

Two chopped parsley

Four chopped green onions

13 chopped mint leaves

Salt to taste

4 tbsp extra virgin olive oil

4 tbsp lime juice

Romaine lettuce leaves to garnishing

Directions :

Soak bulgur for 10 minutes in water.

Drain to remove all the excess water and keep it aside.

Now, mix all the ingredients in a large salad bowl and place them for 30 minutes in the refrigerator to get the best results.

Nutrition Info: Calories: 190 kcal Fat: 10 g Protein: 3.2 g Carbs: 25.5 g Fiber: 3.1 g

Watermelon salad

Preparation time: 15 minutes

Cooking time: 0 minute

Servings: 6

Ingredients:

Honey Vinaigrette

2 tbsp extra virgin olive oil

2 tbsp honey

One pinch of salt

½ chopped watermelon

Watermelon Salad

2 tbsp lime juice

One chopped English cucumber

15 chopped basil leaves

15 chopped mint leaves

½ cup feta cheese

Directions : In a bowl, combine watermelon, herbs, and cucumber and set aside.

In another bowl, mix oil, salt, honey, and lemon juice and pour the dressing into a watermelon bowl.

Toss well and serve.

Nutrition Info: Calories: 192 kcal Fat: 5.6 g Protein: 4.3 g Carbs: 35.9 g Fiber: 11 g

Loaded chickpea salad

Preparation time: 20 minutes

Cooking time: 10 minutes

Servings: 6

Ingredients:

Olive oil

One sliced eggplant

1 cup cooked chickpeas

Three diced Roma tomatoes

3 tbsp Za'atar spice

Salt to taste

½ chopped English cucumber

1 cup chopped parsley

One chopped small red onion

1 cup chopped dill

Garlic Vinaigrette

Two chopped garlic cloves

1/3 cup extra virgin olive oil

2 tbsp lime juice

Salt to taste

Black pepper to taste

Directions :

Season eggplant with salt and set aside for 30 minutes.

Dry eggplant and cook in olive oil for five minutes from each side.

When the eggplant has turned brown from both sides, remove the pan from the flame and keep it aside.

In a bowl, combine cucumber, onions, tomatoes, dill, zaatar, chickpeas, parsley, and mix well.

Place all the dressing ingredients in a bowl and toss well.

Transfer cooked eggplant and chickpeas mixture in one large bowl and poured the dressing over them.

Serve and enjoy it.

Nutrition Info: Calories: 308 kcal Fat: 15.3 g Protein: 11.1 g Carbs: 17.3 g Fiber: 9.6 g

Baba ganoush

Preparation time: 10 minutes

Cooking time: 40 minutes

Servings: 4

Ingredients:

One eggplant

1 tbsp Greek yogurt

olive oil

1.5 tbsp tahini paste

1 tbsp lime juice

One garlic clove

Salt to taste

1 tsp cayenne pepper

Pepper to taste

½ tsp sumac for garnishing

Parsley leaves for garnishing

Toasted pine nuts for garnishing

Directions :

Make slits in eggplant's skin.

Place eggplant skin side upwards in a baking tray.

Spray olive oil over eggplant.

Bake in a preheated oven at 425 degrees for 40 minutes.

Scoop the inner flesh of eggplant out and shift in a food processor. Add garlic, cayenne, yogurt, lime juice, salt, tahini, sumac, pepper, and blend. The baba ganoush is ready.

You can refrigerator for better results for 60 minutes and sprinkle oil, sumac, parsley, and nuts and serve.

Nutrition Info: Calories: 114 kcal Fat: 7.7 g Protein: 2.8 g Carbs: 11.1 g Fiber: 5 g

Salmon fish sticks

Preparation time: 10 minutes

Cooking time: 18 minutes

Servings: 4

Ingredients:

Fish Sticks

2 lb salmon fillet

1/4 tsp salt

1/4 tsp black pepper

First coating

1/2 tsp garlic powder

1/2 tsp dried thyme

1 cup almond meal

1/2 tsp sea salt

1/4 tsp black pepper

Second coating

1/2 tsp salt

2/3 cup chickpea flour

Third coating

Two eggs

Dipping Sauce

1/4 tsp salt

1/4 cup Greek yogurt

1 tsp lemon juice

1 tbsp Dijon mustard

1/2 tsp dill

1/8 tsp garlic powder

Directions : Whisk all the ingredients for the dipping sauce list in a bowl and set aside. The dipping sauce is ready.

Mix garlic, thyme, and almond meal in a bowl. The first coating is ready.

Add chickpea flour in another bowl. The second coating is ready.

Beat the eggs in another bowl. Set aside.

Sprinkle pepper and salt over sliced fish with removed skin.

First, coat the fish with chickpea flour, followed by coating with egg and almond meal coating.

Aline coated fish pieces in a baking sheet covered with parchment paper.

Bake in a preheated oven at 400 degrees for 18 minutes.

Serve baked fish with dipping sauce and serve.

Nutrition Info: Calories: 92 kcal Fat: 5.7 g Protein: 14.4 g Carbs: 4.5 g Fiber: 1.3 g

Baked falafel

Preparation time: 10 minutes

Cooking time: 24 minutes

Servings: 15 patties

Ingredients:

15 oz chickpeas

Three cloves garlic

1/4 cup chopped onion

1/2 cup parsley

2 tsp lemon juice

1/2 tsp baking soda

1 tbsp olive oil

1 tsp ground cumin

3/4 tsp salt

1 tsp coriander

One pinch of cayenne

3 tbsp oat flour

Directions :

Blend all the ingredients except oat flour and baking soda in a food processor to get roughly a blended mixture.

Transfer the mixture to a bowl and add oat flour and baking soda. Using hands, mix the dough well.

Make patties out of the falafel mixture and set aside for 15 minutes.

Bake the falafel patties in a preheated oven at 375 degrees for 12 minutes and serve.

Nutrition Info: Calories: 143 kcal Fat: 5 g Protein: 6 g Carbs: 24 g Fiber: 6 g

Chia Greek yogurt pudding

Preparation time: 10 minutes

Cooking time: 0 minute

Servings: 4

Ingredients:

3/4 cup milk

11 oz f Vanilla Yogurt

2 tbsp pure maple syrup

1 tsp vanilla extract

1/8 tsp salt

1/4 cup chia seeds

Sliced almonds for garnishing

Directions : Whisk all the ingredients in a large bowl. Set aside for 24 hours in the refrigerator.

Mix the mixture gently after 24 hours and serve after garnishing.

Nutrition Info: Calories: 179 kcal Fat: 5.6 g Protein: 10.1 g Carbs: 22.3 g Fiber: 6 g

Air fryer potato wedges

Preparation time: 5 minutes

Cooking time: 30 minutes

Servings: 4

Ingredients:

Two wedges cut potatoes

½ tsp salt

½ tsp paprika

1.5 tbsp olive oil

½ tsp chili powder

1/8 black pepper

Directions : Combine all the ingredients in a bowl. Transfer the mixture to an air fryer basket and cook in a preheated air fryer at 400 degrees for eight minutes from both sides.

Serve and enjoy it.

Nutrition Info: Calories: 129 kcal Fat: g Protein: 2.3 g Carbs: 19 g Fiber: 11 g

Greek-style potatoes

Preparation time: 20 minutes

Cooking time: 120 minutes

Servings: 4

Ingredients:

1/3 cup olive oil

Two chopped garlic cloves

1.5 cups water

Black pepper to taste

¼ cup lemon juice

1 tsp rosemary

1 tsp thyme

Two chicken bouillon cubes

Six chopped potatoes

Directions : Mix all the ingredients in a large bowl and pour over the potatoes placed in the baking tray.

Bake in a preheated oven at 350 degrees for 90 minutes.

Serve and enjoy it.

Nutrition Info: Calories: 418 kcal Fat: 18.5 g Protein: 7 g Carbs: 58.6 g Fiber: 9 g

Skinny slow cooker kale and turkey meatball soup

Preparation time: 15 minutes

Cooking time: 240 minutes

Servings: 4

Ingredients:

¼ cup milk

1 lb lean turkey

Two slices of bread

One chopped shallot

½ tsp grated nutmeg

Two chopped garlic cloves

1 tsp oregano

Kosher salt to taste

1/4 tsp red pepper flakes

Black pepper to taste

2 tbsp chopped parsley

½ cup grated Parmigiano-Reggiano

One egg

8 cups chicken broth

1 tbsp olive oil

15 oz white beans

½ chopped onion

Two sliced carrots

4 cups kale

Directions :

Soak pieces of bread in milk in a bowl followed by the addition of nutmeg, flakes, cheese, turkey, parsley, shallot, oregano, salt, egg, garlic, and pepper.

Mix well using hands. Make meatballs out of the turkey mixture. Fry meatballs in heat olive oil in a skillet over a high flame. Keep the fried meatballs aside for a few minutes.

Place beans, onions, carrot, kale, and broth in a slow cooker, followed by adding meatballs in broth.

Cover the cooker and cook for four hours.

Garnish with grated cheese, parsley, and flakes and serve.

Nutrition Info: Calories: 297 kcal Fat: 10 g Protein: 21 g Carbs: 27 g Fiber: 2 g

Chicken Caprese sandwich

Preparation time: 10 minutes

Cooking time: 6 minutes

Servings: 4

Ingredients:

4 tbsp olive oil

1 tbsp lemon juice

¼ cup basil leaves

1 tsp minced parsley

Kosher salt to taste

Two boneless chicken breasts

Black pepper to taste

10 oz sliced sourdough bread

Eleven Campari tomatoes

8 oz sliced mozzarella cheese

Balsamic vinegar as required

Directions : Add chicken pieces, olive oil, lemon juice, salt, parsley, and pepper in a bowl. Toss well to coat chicken evenly. Set aside.

Grill the chicken on a preheated grill on a medium flame for six minutes from both sides.

Toast the bread drizzled with olive oil.

Sliced the bread into three pieces.

Place chicken pieces, cheese, and tomato slices over each slice of bread.

Sprinkle vinegar, oil, salt, basil, and pepper over the bread slices and serve.

Nutrition Info: Calories: 612.73 kcal Fat: 32.06 g Protein: 34.4 g Carbs: 46.88 g Fiber: 2.25 g

Minestrone

Preparation time: 15 minutes

Cooking time: 30 minutes

Servings: 6

Ingredients:

2 tbsp olive oil

1/3 cup shredded parmesan cheese

Four chopped garlic cloves

One chopped onion

Two chopped celery stalks

1/3 lb green beans

One diced carrot

1 tsp oregano

Salt to taste

1 tsp basil

Black pepper to taste

14 oz crushed tomatoes

28 oz diced tomatoes

6 cups chicken stock

1 cup elbow pasta

15 oz beans

2 tbsp chopped basil

Directions :

Sauté onions in heated olive oil over medium flame for five minutes.

Stir in garlic and cook for half a minute.

Mix carrot and celery and cook for five more minutes with occasional stirring.

Add oregano, beans, salt, basil, and black pepper and cook for another three minutes with constant stirring.

Pour broth followed by the addition of tomatoes and let it boil.

Lower the flame to low and let it simmer for ten minutes.

Add pasta and kidney beans and cook for another ten minutes.

Mix salt and serve after garnishing with cheese and bail.

Nutrition Info: Calories: 260 kcal Fat: 8 g Protein: 15 g Carbs: 37 g Fiber: 10 g

Avocado Caprese wrap

Preparation time: 20 minutes

Cooking time: 0 minute

Servings: 3

Ingredients:

Two tortillas

Balsamic vinegar as needed

One ball mozzarella cheese grated

1/2 cup arugula leaves

One sliced tomato

2 tbsp basil leaves

Kosher salt to taste

One sliced avocado

Olive oil as required

Black pepper to taste

Directions : Place tomato slices and cheese, followed by avocado and basil. Over one side of the tortilla. Pour olive oil and vinegar. Drizzle pepper and salt.

Wrap the tortilla and serve.

Nutrition Info: Calories: 791 kcal Fat: 47 g Protein: 23 g Carbs: 71 g Fiber: 16 g

Avocado and Greek yogurt chicken salad

Preparation time: 10 minutes

Cooking time: 0 minute

Servings: 4

Ingredients:

1 cup plain yogurt

1 tbsp lemon juice

One mashed avocado

1/3 cup dried cranberries

Kosher salt to taste

2 cups shredded chicken

Black pepper to taste

3/4 cup chopped celery

1/3 cup chopped pecans

1/2 cup chopped red grapes

1/3 cup chopped red onion

2 tbsp chopped tarragon

Directions : Whisk all the ingredients in a large mixing bowl. Serve as a salad and enjoy it.

Nutrition Info: Calories: 359 kcal Fat: 19 g Protein: 27 g Carbs: 23 g Fiber: 6 g